The Complete Diabetic Cookbook for Women

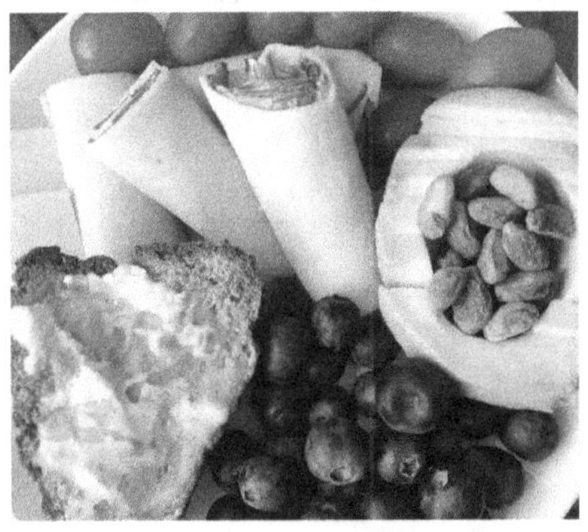

180 Simple, Delicious Recipes to Help You Balance Your Blood Sugar Level

By
Dovie Betty

Table of Content

Introduction

Step into a place where the magic of your cooking does more than satiate hunger—it empowers your health. This book, "The Complete Diabetic Cookbook for Women," is crafted just for you, a sanctuary where every recipe not only delights your palate but also celebrates your health and tenacity in the face of diabetes.

Within these pages, you'll find more than mere meals. These are beacons of light, guiding you to combine taste with health and pleasure with nutrition. Learn how to infuse your diet with balance and joy, accommodating the unique hormonal fluctuations that shape your experience with diabetes.

Consider this book more than a culinary guide—it's a trusted friend. It offers you recipes for energizing breakfasts, sustaining lunches, comforting dinners, and sensible yet indulgent desserts. Rest assured that every dish has been selected with your nutritional needs in mind, ensuring you don't have to sacrifice flavor for your health.

As you embark on this journey, you're not just nourishing your body; you're embracing a lifestyle.

This isn't just about eating well—it's about enriching your life with contentment and healthy choices in the face of diabetes.

Approach this adventure with eagerness and commitment. With each recipe you try and enjoy, you're taking control of diabetic-friendly eating, all while treating yourself with the respect and attention you deserve.

Welcome to a space where your kitchen becomes a haven, a place where wisdom, well-being, and deliciousness are woven into the fabric of your everyday life. Here, let's celebrate and rediscover the joy of cooking, knowing that each meal you prepare is an essential chapter in your story of health and empowerment.

Chapter 1: Understanding Diabetes in Women

Step into the pages of "The Complete Diabetic Cookbook for Women," and you'll gain keen insight into managing diabetes that's tailored specifically to your needs. Recognizing the intricate dance your body performs, the cookbook considers how hormonal fluctuations uniquely influence your blood glucose control differently than they would in men.

As you explore each section, you'll find the content specifically formulated for the female body's natural rhythm—it's a resource designed with you in mind. The cookbook offers not just recipes but wisdom on how to navigate the varying insulin sensitivities brought on by your menstrual cycle, advocating for an adaptable dietary strategy.

With practical guidance, the book equips you to seamlessly sync meal choices with your body's cues, thus stabilizing your blood sugar. The recipes provided support you through hormonal shifts, whether it's by boosting your morning energy or ensuring a steady glucose level during dinner. These culinary plans also serve as a lesson in dietary autonomy—teaching you to make savvy decisions about quantities, healthier ingredient swaps, and deciphering the complexities of glycemic indices.

More than a collection of meal ideas, it's an approach to eating that celebrates your femininity and diabetic health, designed to be both intuitive and personalized just for you.

Types of Diabetes

You're dealing with a life-long condition called diabetes, which comes in several forms, each affecting how your body deals with blood sugar.
If you have type 1 diabetes, your body's immune system, by mistake, attacks the cells making insulin in your pancreas. This kind usually kicks in during your youth and means you'll need to take insulin daily because your body can't make it anymore.
If you're facing Type 2 diabetes, your body isn't using insulin the way it should, often because of factors like your weight, how active you are, and your genes. You might manage this type with

lifestyle changes and medications, and sometimes you'll need insulin as well.

During pregnancy, you might get what's known as gestational diabetes, which happens when pregnancy hormones cause your blood sugar to rise. It's temporary, but keep an eye out since it could increase your chance of developing type 2 diabetes later on.

There are also rarer types, like monogenic diabetes, caused by gene changes, and diabetes that sometimes comes with cystic fibrosis.

Unique Aspects of Diabetes in Women

Diabetes affects you as a woman in specific ways that differ from men. Your hormonal variations make controlling your blood sugar more complex, especially during your menstrual cycle, when levels can fluctuate significantly. It's smart to check your glucose often during these periods.

If you're planning a pregnancy or become pregnant, it's crucial to manage your diabetes vigilantly to protect both you and your baby from the risks associated with gestational diabetes. You'll likely need to fine-tune your diabetes management strategy in collaboration with your healthcare team.

As you approach menopause, the challenge continues as it can cause further irregularities in your blood sugar levels, emphasizing the need for meticulous monitoring and diet control.

In your resource, "The Complete Diabetic Cookbook for Women," the meals and strategies are created with an understanding of these hormonal changes. It presents you with wholesome, tasty recipes that aim to keep your blood sugar steady, featuring nutrient-dense foods that suit a woman's needs and have a minimal impact on your blood sugar. This practical guidance is formulated to support your distinctive health needs as a woman with diabetes.

The Role of Hormones

Hormones are key players in "The Complete Diabetic Cookbook for Women," profoundly impacting how you manage your blood sugar. Think of hormones as tiny communicators circulating in your body, instructing various parts on when to spring into action. As a woman, your life stages—like your menstrual cycle, pregnancy, and menopause—introduce hormonal changes that influence diabetes management uniquely compared to men.

Your menstrual cycle causes hormone levels to swing, which, in turn, swings your blood sugar levels. The cookbook adapts to this by recommending more frequent glucose checks and tweaks in your diet.

When you're pregnant, maintaining the right hormonal balance is doubly important for both your and your baby's health. The recipes in the cookbook cater to this by focusing on meals that help keep your blood sugar levels steady, directly addressing the challenge of gestational diabetes.

With menopause comes a fresh set of hormonal adjustments that can unsettle your blood sugar control. The cookbook offers nutritional strategies to help smooth out these changes.

Each recipe and piece of advice in the cookbook is tailored to support you, adapting to your body's hormonal changes, to aid in your journey as a woman managing diabetes.

Symptoms and Diagnosis

Symptoms and Diagnosis in "The Complete Diabetic Cookbook for Women," it talks to you about what to look out for: increased thirst, the need to urinate more often, feeling incredibly tired, and not seeing as clearly as usual. These symptoms are not just everyday tiredness; they could be warning signs of diabetes, something you shouldn't ignore.

The cookbook suggests that you see your doctor for a definitive diagnosis, with a blood test as the likely next step. You might have the Fasting Plasma Glucose Test, the Oral Glucose Tolerance Test, or the A1C Test, all of which assess your blood sugar levels and how your body manages glucose.

It also reminds you to trust what your body tells you. Do you squint to read recipes or constantly interrupt cooking to use the bathroom? These personal experiences are vital pieces of information that, along with a doctor's advice, will help diagnose your condition accurately.

By recognizing these symptoms and understanding how to get diagnosed, you take control. You can then fully utilize the cookbook's nutritious recipes to regulate your blood sugar and lead a healthier lifestyle.

Chapter 2: Causes and Risk Factors

As you age, especially past 45, you should pay closer attention to signs of diabetes. An inactive lifestyle or a diet filled with processed foods and sugar can lead to insulin resistance, which boosts your diabetes risk.

The cookbook also highlights that, as a woman, you face unique risks such as polycystic ovary syndrome (PCOS) and the possibility of developing diabetes during pregnancy. These health issues can make you more susceptible to type 2 diabetes later on.

With these insights, you'll be guided to reflect on your lifestyle habits. Using the recipes and advice from the cookbook, you can actively work to lower your risk and take control of your health.

Lifestyle and Environmental Factors

In "The Complete Diabetic Cookbook for Women," there's a crucial piece that talks to you about how your daily choices and where you live and work can affect your chances of developing diabetes. Take a look around you. Are you surrounded by fast food and sugary snacks? This book will push you to rethink these spaces—your kitchen, your job, even where you hang out with friends. It's about the environment shaping your food and exercise habits. You are in control of your life choices, like what you eat and how much you move. This cookbook offers straightforward advice: pick whole foods that are packed with nutrients and make exercise a regular part of your life to keep your blood sugar levels stable.

It gives you tips for making healthy eating and enjoyable physical activity a natural part of your day-to-day. It's not about short-term fixes; it's about long-term changes. By understanding and tweaking your surroundings and routines, as recommended by this cookbook, you'll pave the way for better diabetes management and improved overall wellness.

Gestational Diabetes Insight

In the women's diabetic cookbook you'll find, there's a handy part about gestational diabetes, which you might face while pregnant. It's when your blood sugar goes high, which wasn't an issue before you got pregnant. It's really important because it can affect both you and your baby's health.

The book will show you ways to handle gestational diabetes well. It'll be key for you to check your blood sugar often to keep track of your health. What you eat is super important, and the book will guide you to have a good mix of protein, carbs, and fats. You'll be eating more foods full of fiber, like whole grains, beans, and veggies.

Staying active is another big help, as moving around can keep your blood sugar in check and make your pregnancy healthier. The cookbook will make sure you've got tasty recipes that are right for your health. By following the book's advice, you can look after yourself and get ready for your baby to arrive healthy and happy.

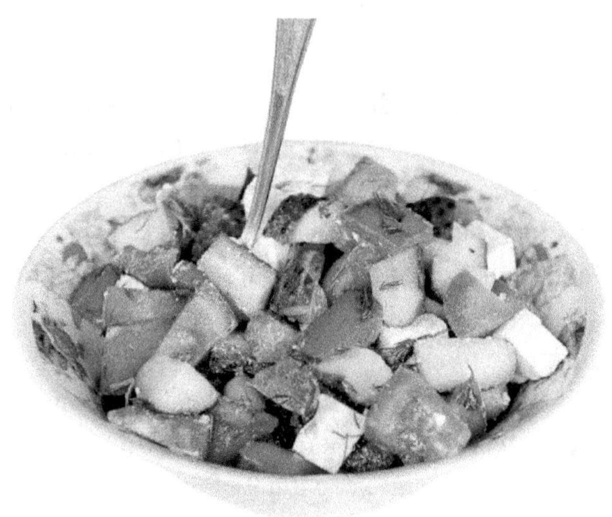

Chapter 3: Diabetes Prevention Strategies

"The Complete Diabetic Cookbook for Women" equips you with key strategies for dodging diabetes. Prioritize unrefined, natural foods—vibrant veggies, quality proteins, and intact grains—to keep your blood sugar balanced; they're your defense line.

The cookbook acts as a mentor, introducing you to portion control as a vital tactic to curtail overeating that could escalate your risk. You'll learn to gauge portions with ease, crafting well-rounded meals that are hearty but not overindulgent.

Physical activity isn't just a suggestion; it's a vital part of your routine. The book advocates for consistent, enjoyable exercise that enhances your body's insulin response and aids in weight management.

But it goes beyond diet and exercise; staying hydrated and getting proper sleep are crucial too, influencing your metabolism and hunger levels.

Fundamentally, this cookbook isn't confined to meal prep; it's a holistic approach to a lifestyle that steers clear of diabetes. It equips you with the know-how to make choices that build a fortress against the disease.

Nutritional Guidelines

"The Complete Diabetic Cookbook for Women" equips you with nutritional advice to help ward off diabetes. Embrace a diet centered on whole, unprocessed foods. Load up on vibrant veggies that are both low in calories and packed with fiber—they'll keep you full without causing blood sugar levels to rise. Choose lean proteins to preserve muscle and keep you feeling satisfied, all while steering clear of unhealthy fats. Whole grains are essential, too; they give you lasting energy and the fiber needed for steady blood sugar control.

Understanding portion sizes is also vital; it's about knowing just the right amount your body needs. Use visual comparisons to help; for instance, your protein serving should be no larger than your own palm.

Adding exercise to your daily routine is important as well; it increases your body's sensitivity to insulin, which improves blood sugar management. Find physical activities you enjoy, whether that's a fast-paced walk, dancing, or yoga, to seamlessly integrate exercise into your life.

Remember that staying hydrated by drinking water helps control your appetite, and getting plenty of sleep is crucial for keeping hunger-related hormones in check.

These guidelines are less about rapid transformations and more about long-term lifestyle changes. Let this cookbook be more than a collection of recipes; let it serve as a day-to-day guide for making choices that bolster your defense against diabetes with practicality and ease.

Physical Activity for Prevention

In the "Diabetes Prevention Strategies" section of "The Complete Diabetic Cookbook for Women," there's a key focus on how important it is for you to weave exercise into your daily life. It's not about grueling gym sessions; it's about finding joy in being more active. This approach boosts your body's ability to regulate sugar levels and reduces your risk of developing diabetes.

Picture this: your exercise isn't a separate, time-consuming task. It's about smart choices like taking the stairs, parking further away when you run errands, or fitting in quick walks throughout your day. Small changes like these can have big impacts on your health.

Selecting an activity you enjoy ensures you'll stick with it. Maybe that's a fast walk in the park, a fun dance class, or relaxing yoga – whatever gets you moving and you can enjoy regularly. It's the regularity that's vital, not how tough the workout is. Combining this approach with the healthy eating tips from the cookbook creates a solid defense system for your body, helping you prevent type 2 diabetes by living an active, healthy life.

Chapter 4: The Healing Kitchen

"The Healing Kitchen" from "The Complete Diabetic Cookbook for Women," you transform your kitchen into a battleground against diabetes. This chapter teaches you to prepare foods that do more than just satiate your hunger. They are instrumental in keeping your blood sugar levels balanced, which is key to managing and warding off diabetes.

Visualize your kitchen not just as a place for meals but as your personal wellness sanctuary. You'll be choosing ingredients like whole grains, colorful veggies, and lean protein—all carefully picked for their role in stabilizing glucose levels and aiding you in maintaining a healthy weight.

Your seasoning cabinet is no longer for flavor alone. You'll learn to select spices that offer flavor plus health benefits, such as the anti-inflammatory properties of cinnamon, which reduce diabetes-related inflammation.

Considering it's designed with women in mind, every recipe within "The Healing Kitchen" caters to your active life. Whether it's a quick bite, a satisfying main dish, or even a luscious treat suitable for a diabetic diet, all are straightforward and easy to prepare.

Look at every dish you create as a positive step towards a healthier self. This chapter is more than mere recipes—it represents a significant era of your life where you harness culinary power for healing, taking control against diabetes with smart nutrition choices.

Essential Nutrients for Diabetic Health

In the "Healing Kitchen" section of "The Complete Diabetic Cookbook for Women," the focus is on crucial nutrients that are a must for managing your diabetes. Fiber is a hero here; it helps pace digestion, keeping blood sugar levels more consistent. You'll be incorporating a lot of veggies, seeds, and whole grains to make this happen.

Healthy fats shouldn't be feared but rather welcomed. They are friends of your heart and don't mess with your glucose. Avocadoes, nuts, and olive oil will be your go-to for meals that satisfy and protect your health.

Lean proteins—think chicken, legumes, and fish—are your muscle-repairing, hunger-satisfying saviors that don't cause sugar levels to surge. They'll be your regular energy source.

Complex carbs will also form a key part of your diet. They're the kinds that nourish and release sugar slowly and steadily, like quinoa and sweet potatoes, so there are no sudden sugar spikes.

Antioxidants and magnesium aren't just buzzwords; they're practical additions to your diet. Berries, dark chocolate, leafy greens, and nuts come into play here, supporting your body's insulin function and shielding your cells from damage.

This isn't just theoretical nutrition—it's about concrete choices you make daily in your kitchen. "The Healing Kitchen" transforms nutritional science into simple meal choices, giving you the power to handle your diabetes with ease and delight.

Foods to Embrace

In "The Complete Diabetic Cookbook for Women," "The Healing Kitchen" section guides you to foods that will aid in controlling your diabetes.

Start with fiber-rich choices—vegetables, seeds, and grains like leafy greens, chia, and brown rice. They don't just fill you up; they stabilize your blood sugar and aid in digestion.

Incorporate good fats into your diet. Avocado, nuts, and olive oil aren't just flavor enhancements; they're vital for maintaining a healthy heart and balancing your glucose levels.

Proteins should be lean, like turkey, beans, and fish. They do more than satisfy your hunger; they repair muscles and help you stay full, keeping blood sugar levels steady.

Choose complex carbohydrates for energy that lasts without a rapid sugar increase. Foods like whole wheat pasta and butternut squash are your friends.

Don't forget foods high in antioxidants and magnesium. Blueberries, dark leafy greens, and nuts aren't just treats; they improve insulin function and protect your cells.

These suggested foods are practical tools in your diabetes management—they're not just good on paper. Introduce them into your daily meals to manage your condition deliciously and effectively.

Foods to Avoid

In "The Healing Kitchen" from "The Complete Diabetic Cookbook for Women," you're advised to be cautious with your food choices to manage your diabetes effectively.

Steer clear of sweet drinks like sodas and juice with added sugars. These can cause your blood sugar levels to rise rapidly. Water or herbal teas are safer options to keep you hydrated without the added sugar.

Avoid white bread and other refined carbs that lack nutrients and cause blood sugar levels to rise and fall quickly. Instead, go for whole grains, such as brown rice or oats, which provide more stable energy.

Processed meats, including sausages and deli slices, should be off your list. They're loaded with sodium and unhealthy additives. Pick healthier proteins, such as baked fish or skinless poultry, to keep blood sugar in check.

Stay away from trans fats found in some processed snacks and spreads; these fats can harm your heart and reduce insulin sensitivity. Always check food labels and incorporate fats that are good for you, such as those found in nuts or olive oil.

Lastly, minimize full-fat dairy products that can affect your heart health. Opt for low-fat dairy or consider plant-based alternatives in moderation.

Remember, from "The Complete Diabetic Cookbook for Women," by choosing wisely and avoiding these foods, you're not just controlling your blood sugar; you're boosting your overall well-being.

Chapter 5: Customizing Your Meal Plan

Meal Planning for Diabetic

Meal planning for diabetes management involves allocating specific times and macronutrients (carbohydrates, proteins, and fats) to ensure blood glucose levels remain stable throughout the day. Here's how to approach it, followed by its benefits:

Steps for Meal Planning:

1. Carbohydrate Counting: Keep track of the carbs in each meal, as they have the most significant effect on blood sugar. Choose high-fiber, low-glycemic index foods like whole grains, legumes, and non-starchy vegetables.

2. Meal Timing: Eat at regular times each day to help regulate blood sugar. This can prevent spikes and dips in glucose levels.

3. Portion Sizes: Monitor portions to avoid overeating, which can lead to increased blood sugar.

4. Balanced Meals: Include a mix of carbohydrates, proteins, and fats to slow digestion and the absorption of sugar.

5. Hydration: Drink water to help manage blood sugar levels and overall health.

6. Variety: Incorporate a variety of foods to meet all nutritional requirements without becoming monotonous.

Benefits:

1. Improved Blood Sugar Control:

Regular, balanced meals can prevent spikes in blood sugar and help manage A1C levels.

2. Weight Management: By controlling portion sizes and avoiding high-calorie foods, individuals can maintain a healthy weight which is crucial in diabetes management.

3. Lower Risk of Complications:

Consistent blood sugar levels can reduce the risk of complications such as neuropathy, retinopathy, and cardiovascular disease.

4. Energy Balance: A consistent meal schedule can help maintain energy levels throughout the day.

5. Healthy Eating Habits: Meal planning encourages a healthier relationship with food, and can lead to better food choices.

6. Reduced Stress and Anxiety: Knowing what and when you're going to eat reduces decision fatigue and the stress of managing diabetes.

7. Better Overall Health: By meeting nutritional needs, planning meals helps support the immune system and overall well-being.

Proper meal planning is a cornerstone of diabetes management, leading to improved health outcomes and quality of life. Always consult with a healthcare provider or dietitian when creating a meal plan for diabetes.

Diabetes Meal Plan

Day 1:
- Breakfast: Scrambled eggs with spinach and whole-grain toast.
- Lunch: Grilled chicken salad with mixed greens, tomatoes, cucumbers, and a vinaigrette dressing.
- Dinner: Baked salmon with steamed broccoli and quinoa.
- Snacks: Greek yogurt and a handful of almonds.
Day 2:
- Breakfast: Greek yogurt with mixed berries and a sprinkle of chia seeds.
- Lunch: Turkey and avocado wrap in a whole-grain tortilla with mixed veggies on the side.
- Dinner: Stir-fried tofu with mixed vegetables over brown rice.
- Snacks: Sliced apple with peanut butter.
Day 3:

- Breakfast: Oatmeal topped with sliced strawberries and a dash of cinnamon.
- Lunch: Lentil soup with a side of whole-grain bread.
- Dinner: Grilled lean steak with roasted sweet potatoes and green beans.
- Snacks: Raw veggies (carrot, cucumber) with hummus.

Day 4:
- Breakfast: Cottage cheese with pineapple chunks and flaxseeds.
- Lunch: Quinoa salad with chickpeas, spinach, and feta cheese.
- Dinner: Boneless chicken breast with Mediterranean salsa, and a side of couscous.
- Snacks: A small peach and a few walnuts.

Day 5:
- Breakfast: Spinach and mushroom omelet.
- Lunch: Tuna salad stuffed in a tomato with a side of mixed greens.
- Dinner: Turkey chili with a variety of beans and a small whole-grain roll.
- Snacks: A small pear and a string cheese.

Day 6:
- Breakfast: Smoothie with spinach, protein powder, half a banana, and almond milk.
- Lunch: Chicken Caesar salad with a light Caesar dressing and whole-grain croutons.

- Dinner: Baked cod with a light lemon-dill sauce, asparagus, and wild rice.
- Snacks: Mixed nuts and blueberries.
Day 7:
- **Breakfast: Whole-grain waffles with a light spread of almond butter and sugar-free syrup.
- Lunch: Black bean soup with a small side salad.
- Dinner: Pork tenderloin with a small baked potato and roasted brussel sprouts.
- Snacks: Sliced bell peppers with a low-fat ranch dip.
General Tips:
- Monitor carbohydrate intake to help regulate blood sugar.
- Choose whole-grain or whole-food starches over processed ones for better nutrient intake and improved blood sugar control.
- Prioritize lean proteins to help with satiety and maintain muscle mass.
- Include a variety of non-starchy vegetables for fiber, vitamins, and minerals.
- Moderate the intake of fats, focusing on sources of healthy fats such as avocados, nuts, and olive oil.
- Stay hydrated and minimize the intake of sugary beverages.

Shopping list

1. Whole Grains:
   - Brown Rice: Rich in fiber, it helps in blood sugar control.
   - Quinoa: Contains protein and fiber, beneficial for blood sugar management.
2. Non-Starchy Vegetables:
   - Broccoli: High in fiber and low in calories.
   - Spinach: Nutrient-dense and low in carbohydrates.
3. Fresh Fruits (in moderation):
   - Berries: Antioxidant-rich and relatively low in sugar.
   - Apples: Provide fiber and vitamin C.
4. Lean Proteins:
   - Chicken Breast: A good source of protein without the high fat.
   - Turkey: Another lean protein choice, ideal for controlling fat intake.
5. Seafood:
   - Salmon: Rich in omega-3 fatty acids and protein.
   - Tuna: Offers protein and is heart-healthy.
6. Legumes:

- Lentils: High in fiber and protein, great for blood sugar stability.

- Chickpeas: Can be included in variety of dishes for added fiber and protein.

7. Healthy Fats:

- Avocado: Contains monounsaturated fats which are heart-healthy.

- Nuts: Almonds, walnuts, and pecans are great sources of healthy fats and fiber.

8. Dairy or Alternatives:

- Low-Fat Greek Yogurt: High in protein and calcium.

- Almond Milk (unsweetened): A non-dairy alternative with lower carbs.

9. Cooking Oils:

- Olive Oil: Source of healthy monounsaturated fats.

- Canola Oil: Low in saturated fats and has a neutral flavor.

10. Herbs and Spices:

- Cinnamon: Can help lower blood sugar levels.

- Turmeric: Has anti-inflammatory properties.

- Garlic: Adds flavor without adding sodium.

11. Eggs:

- A versatile source of high-quality protein.

12. Vinegar:

- Apple Cider Vinegar: May help with glycemic control.

13. Seeds:

- Chia Seeds: High in fiber and omega-3 fatty acids.

  - Flaxseeds: Another good source of omega-3s and fiber.

14. Whole Grain Flours:

  - Almond Flour: Low in carbohydrates and high in healthy fats.

  - Coconut Flour: High in fiber and low in carbs.

15. Sweeteners:

  - Stevia: A natural sweetener with no carbohydrates.

  - Erythritol: Low-calorie sugar alcohol that doesn't spike blood sugar.

16. Condiments:

  - Mustard: Low in calories and carbs.

  - Salsa: Make sure it's sugar-free.

17. Canned Goods:

  - Diced Tomatoes: Look for versions with no added sugar or salt.

  - Black Beans: Rinse thoroughly to reduce sodium.

18. Frozen Produce:

  - Mixed Berries: Convenient for smoothies or toppings.

  - Stir-fry Veggies: Quick and easy to add to meals.

19. Beverages:

  - Green Tea: Antioxidant-rich and calorie-free.

  - Sparkling Water: A fizzy, hydrating option without sugar.

20. Snacking Options:

- Popcorn (unsalted, air-popped): A low calorie, high fiber snack.

- Edamame: A good source of protein and fiber to satisfy cravings.

Incorporating these ingredients into your shopping list can lead to a diverse, balanced diet that supports diabetic health and overall well-being.

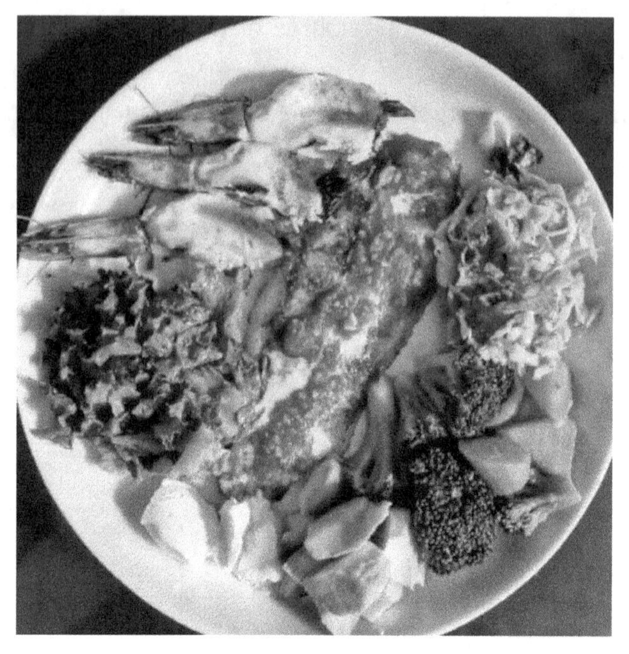

Chapter 6: Recipes for Healthy Living

Step into your kitchen sanctuary with the "Recipes for Healthy Living" section from "The Complete Diabetic Cookbook for Women." Here, discover recipes that cater to your taste and health, all tailored to make managing diabetes simple and enjoyable. Every meal is a balance of deliciousness and nutrition, perfect for your dynamic life. This chapter is your ally, ensuring you enjoy wholesome meals that support your wellness journey. Let these recipes inspire a healthier you, transforming the way you eat without sacrificing taste or convenience.

Breakfasts Recipes

1: **Vegetable Omelette:**
Ingredients:2 eggs
1/4 cup diced bell peppers
1/4 cup spinach
1/4 cup tomatoes
Salt and pepper to taste
Nutritional Value: High in protein, low in carbs
Cooking Time: 10 minutes

2: **Greek Yogurt Parfait:**
Ingredients:1/2 cup Greek yogurt
1/4 cup blueberries
1 tablespoon chopped almonds
1 teaspoon honey (optional)
Nutritional Value: Rich in protein and
antioxidants
Cooking Time: 5 minutes

3: **Quinoa Breakfast Bowl:**
Ingredients:1/2 cup cooked quinoa
1/4 cup sliced strawberries
1 tablespoon chia seeds
1 tablespoon almond butter
Nutritional Value: Packed with fiber and protein
Cooking Time: 15 minutes (including quinoa
preparation)

4: **Cottage Cheese Pancakes:**
Ingredients:1/2 cup cottage cheese
2 eggs
2 tablespoons almond flour
1/2 teaspoon vanilla extract
Nutritional Value: Low in carbs, high in protein
Cooking Time: 12 minutes

5: **Avocado and Smoked Salmon Wrap:**
Ingredients:1 whole-grain tortilla
1/2 avocado, sliced
2 ounces smoked salmon
1 tablespoon cream cheese
Nutritional Value: Healthy fats and omega-3
Cooking Time: 5 minutes

6: **Chia Seed Pudding:**
Ingredients:2 tablespoons chia seeds
1/2 cup unsweetened almond milk
1/4 teaspoon vanilla extract
1/2 cup mixed berries
Nutritional Value: High in fiber and omega-3
Cooking Time: 5 minutes (plus refrigeration time)

7: **Sweet Potato Hash Browns:**
Ingredients:1 medium sweet potato, grated
1 tablespoon olive oil
1/4 teaspoon paprika
Salt and pepper to taste
Nutritional Value: Rich in vitamins and fiber
Cooking Time: 15 minutes

8: **Egg Muffins with Vegetables:**
Ingredients:4 eggs
1/4 cup diced bell peppers
1/4 cup spinach
1/4 cup cherry tomatoes, halved
Nutritional Value: High in protein, low in carbs
Cooking Time: 20 minutes

9: **Almond Flour Waffles:**
Ingredients:1 cup almond flour
2 eggs
1/4 cup unsweetened almond milk
1/2 teaspoon baking powder
Nutritional Value: Low in carbs, high in protein
Cooking Time: 10 minutes

10: **Mushroom and Spinach Scramble:**
Ingredients:2 eggs
1/2 cup sliced mushrooms

1 cup baby spinach
1 tablespoon olive oil
Nutritional Value: Rich in vitamins and minerals
Cooking Time: 8 minutes

11: **Egg White Veggie Scramble:**

Ingredients:3 egg whites
1/4 cup diced zucchini
1/4 cup diced bell peppers
1/4 cup diced onions
Salt and pepper to taste
Nutritional Value: Low in calories, high in protein
Cooking Time: 10 minutes

12: **Coconut Flour Pancakes:**

Ingredients:1/4 cup coconut flour
2 eggs
1/2 cup unsweetened almond milk
1/2 teaspoon baking powder
Nutritional Value: Low in carbs, high in fiber
Cooking Time: 8 minutes

13: **Smashed Avocado on Whole Grain Toast:**

Ingredients:1 slice whole grain bread
1/2 avocado, smashed
1 teaspoon lemon juice

Pinch of red pepper flakes
Nutritional Value: Healthy fats and fiber
Cooking Time: 5 minutes

14: **Berry Protein Smoothie:**

Ingredients:1/2 cup mixed berries (strawberries, blueberries, raspberries)

1/2 cup unsweetened almond milk

1 scoop vanilla protein powder

1 tablespoon chia seeds

Nutritional Value: High in antioxidants and protein

Preparation Time: 5 minutes

15: **Turkey and Veggie Breakfast Wrap:**

Ingredients:1 whole-grain tortilla

2 slices turkey breast

1/4 cup diced tomatoes

1/4 cup shredded lettuce

1 tablespoon Greek yogurt (as a spread)

Nutritional Value: Lean protein and fiber

Cooking Time: 7 minutes

16: **Almond Butter Banana Smoothie Bowl:**

Ingredients:1 medium banana, sliced

2 tablespoons almond butter

1/2 cup unsweetened almond milk

1 tablespoon flaxseeds

Nutritional Value: Rich in potassium, healthy fats, and fiber
Preparation Time: 5 minutes

17: **Spinach and Feta Egg Muffins:**

Ingredients:4 eggs
1/2 cup chopped spinach
1/4 cup crumbled feta cheese
Salt and pepper to taste
Nutritional Value: High in protein and iron
Cooking Time: 15 minutes

18: **Chickpea Flour Pancakes:**

Ingredients:1/2 cup chickpea flour
1/2 cup water
1/4 teaspoon cumin powder
1/4 cup diced bell peppers
Nutritional Value: Low in carbs, high in protein and fiber
Cooking Time: 10 minutes

19: **Salmon and Avocado Wrap:**

Ingredients:1 whole-grain tortilla
3 ounces grilled salmon
1/4 avocado, sliced
1 tablespoon plain Greek yogurt
Nutritional Value: Omega-3 fatty acids and protein
Cooking Time: 8 minutes

20: **Cauliflower Hash Browns:**

Ingredients:1 cup grated cauliflower

1 egg

1/4 teaspoon garlic powder

Salt and pepper to taste

Nutritional Value: Low in carbs, high in vitamins

Cooking Time: 12 minutes

21: **Berry and Almond Overnight Oats:**

Ingredients:1/2 cup rolled oats

1/2 cup unsweetened almond milk

1/4 cup mixed berries (strawberries, blueberries)

1 tablespoon almond slices

Nutritional Value: High in fiber and antioxidants

Preparation Time: 5 minutes (overnight soaking)

22: **Mediterranean Frittata:**

Ingredients:4 eggs

1/4 cup diced tomatoes

1/4 cup chopped spinach

2 tablespoons feta cheese

Nutritional Value: Rich in protein and vitamins

Cooking Time: 15 minutes

23: **Peanut Butter Banana Wrap:**
Ingredients:1 whole-grain tortilla
2 tablespoons natural peanut butter
1 medium banana, sliced
Cinnamon for flavor
Nutritional Value: Healthy fats, potassium, and protein
Preparation Time: 5 minutes

24: **Cabbage and Turkey Sausage Skillet:**
Ingredients:1 cup shredded cabbage
2 turkey sausage links, sliced
1/4 cup diced onions
1/4 teaspoon paprika
Nutritional Value: Low in carbs, high in fiber and protein
Cooking Time: 12 minutes

25: **Yogurt and Granola Parfait:**
Ingredients:1/2 cup plain Greek yogurt
1/4 cup granola (unsweetened)
1/4 cup mixed berries
1 tablespoon chopped nuts (e.g., almonds, walnuts)
Nutritional Value: High in protein, fiber, and antioxidants
Preparation Time: 5 minutes

26: **Sweet Potato and Spinach Breakfast** Casserole:
Ingredients:1 medium sweet potato, grated
1 cup fresh spinach, chopped
4 eggs
1/4 cup shredded mozzarella cheese
Nutritional Value: High in fiber, vitamins, and protein
Cooking Time: 25 minutes

27: **Cherry Almond Chia Pudding:**
Ingredients:2 tablespoons chia seeds
1/2 cup unsweetened almond milk
1/4 cup fresh cherries, pitted and chopped
1 tablespoon sliced almonds
Nutritional Value: Rich in omega-3, antioxidants, and fiber
Preparation Time: 5 minutes (plus refrigeration time)

28: **Egg and Veggie Breakfast Burrito:**
Ingredients:2 eggs
1/4 cup black beans, rinsed and drained
1/4 cup diced bell peppers
1 whole-grain tortilla
Nutritional Value: Protein, fiber, and vitamins

Cooking Time: 10 minutes

29: **Cauliflower and Broccoli Egg Muffins:**

Ingredients:4 eggs
1/2 cup cauliflower, finely chopped
1/2 cup broccoli, finely chopped
Salt and pepper to taste
Nutritional Value: Low in carbs, high in fiber and protein
Cooking Time: 18 minutes

30: **Pumpkin Spice Chia Pudding**:

Ingredients:3 tablespoons chia seeds
1/2 cup unsweetened almond milk
2 tablespoons pumpkin puree
1/2 teaspoon pumpkin spice
Nutritional Value: Rich in fiber, vitamins, and omega-3
Preparation Time: 5 minutes (plus refrigeration time)

31: **Cottage Cheese and Pineapple Bowl:**

Ingredients:1/2 cup low-fat cottage cheese
1/2 cup fresh pineapple chunks
1 tablespoon chopped mint leaves
1 tablespoon chopped walnuts

Nutritional Value: High in protein, vitamins, and healthy fats

Preparation Time: 5 minutes

32: **Turmeric and Cinnamon Quinoa Porridge:**

Ingredients:1/2 cup cooked quinoa

1/2 cup unsweetened almond milk

1/4 teaspoon turmeric powder

1/2 teaspoon cinnamon

Nutritional Value: Rich in antioxidants, fiber, and anti-inflammatory properties

Cooking Time: 10 minutes

33: **Egg and Avocado Breakfast Salad:**

Ingredients:2 boiled eggs, sliced

1/2 avocado, diced

1 cup mixed greens (spinach, arugula)

1 tablespoon balsamic vinaigrette

Nutritional Value: High in protein, healthy fats, and vitamins

Preparation Time: 7 minutes

34: **Blueberry and Walnut Oat Bars:**

Ingredients:1 cup rolled oats

1/2 cup blueberries

1/4 cup chopped walnuts

1/4 cup almond butter

Nutritional Value: Fiber, antioxidants, and healthy fats

Cooking Time: 20 minutes

35: **Eggplant and Tomato Breakfast Casserole:**

Ingredients:1 cup eggplant, diced

1 cup cherry tomatoes, halved

3 eggs

1/4 cup feta cheese, crumbled

Nutritional Value: Low in carbs, high in vitamins and protein

Cooking Time: 30 minutes

36: **Mango and Cottage Cheese Parfait:**

Ingredients:1/2 cup low-fat cottage cheese

1/2 cup diced mango

1 tablespoon chopped pistachios

1 teaspoon honey (optional)

Nutritional Value: Protein, vitamins, and healthy fats

Preparation Time: 5 minutes

37: **Chickpea and Spinach Breakfast Bowl:**

Ingredients:1/2 cup canned chickpeas, rinsed and drained

1 cup fresh spinach

1/4 cup cherry tomatoes, halved

1 tablespoon olive oil

Nutritional Value: Fiber, protein, and vitamins

Cooking Time: 10 minutes

38: Peach and Almond Overnight Chia Pudding:

Ingredients:2 tablespoons chia seeds

1/2 cup unsweetened almond milk

1/2 cup diced peaches

1 tablespoon slivered almonds

Nutritional Value: Omega-3, antioxidants, and fiber

Preparation Time: 5 minutes (plus refrigeration time)

39: Cauliflower and Cheese Breakfast Muffins:

Ingredients:2 cups cauliflower, grated

2 eggs

1/4 cup grated cheddar cheese

1/4 teaspoon garlic powder

Nutritional Value: Low in carbs, high in fiber and protein

Cooking Time: 25 minutes

40: Pumpkin and Walnut Smoothie:

Ingredients:1/2 cup canned pumpkin puree

1/2 cup unsweetened almond milk

1/4 cup walnuts

1/2 teaspoon cinnamon

Nutritional Value: Rich in fiber, antioxidants, and omega-3

Preparation Time: 5 minutes

41: **Broccoli and Mushroom Egg Muffins:**

Ingredients:4 eggs

1/2 cup broccoli, finely chopped

1/4 cup mushrooms, diced

Salt and pepper to taste

Nutritional Value: High in protein, low in carbs

Cooking Time: 15 minutes

42: **Apple Cinnamon Chia Seed Pudding:**

Ingredients:2 tablespoons chia seeds

1/2 cup unsweetened almond milk

1/2 apple, diced

1/2 teaspoon cinnamon

Nutritional Value: Rich in fiber, vitamins, and antioxidants

Preparation Time: 5 minutes (plus refrigeration time)

43: **Turkey and Vegetable Breakfast Skillet:**

Ingredients:1/2 cup lean ground turkey
1/4 cup bell peppers, diced
1/4 cup zucchini, sliced
1 tablespoon olive oil
Nutritional Value: High in protein, low in carbs
Cooking Time: 12 minutes

44: **Ricotta and Berry Stuffed French Toast:**

Ingredients:2 slices whole grain bread
1/4 cup ricotta cheese
1/2 cup mixed berries
1 egg
Nutritional Value: Protein, fiber, and antioxidants
Cooking Time: 10 minutes

45: **Tomato and Basil Avocado Toast:**

Ingredients:1 slice whole grain bread
1/2 avocado, mashed
1/2 cup cherry tomatoes, sliced
Fresh basil leaves for garnish
Nutritional Value: Healthy fats, vitamins, and antioxidants
Preparation Time: 5 minutes

46: **Zucchini and Goat Cheese Frittata:**

Ingredients:4 eggs
1/2 cup zucchini, grated
2 tablespoons crumbled goat cheese
Salt and pepper to taste
Nutritional Value: Protein, vitamins, and low in carbs
Cooking Time: 15 minutes

47: **Blueberry Almond Chia Pudding Parfait:**

Ingredients:3 tablespoons chia seeds
1/2 cup unsweetened almond milk
1/4 cup blueberries
1 tablespoon chopped almonds
Nutritional Value: Omega-3, antioxidants, and fiber
Preparation Time: 5 minutes (plus refrigeration time)

48: **Mushroom and Spinach Breakfast Burrito:**

Ingredients:1 whole-grain tortilla
2 eggs, scrambled
1/2 cup mushrooms, sliced
1 cup fresh spinach
Nutritional Value: Protein, fiber, and vitamins
Cooking Time: 10 minutes

49: **Cinnamon Walnut Oatmeal:**

Ingredients:1/2 cup rolled oats

1 cup water

1/4 teaspoon cinnamon

1 tablespoon chopped walnuts

Nutritional Value: Fiber, antioxidants, and healthy fats

Cooking Time: 7 minutes

50:**Salmon and Asparagus Omelette:**

Ingredients:2 eggs

2 ounces smoked salmon

1/4 cup asparagus, chopped

Salt and pepper to taste

Nutritional Value: Omega-3, protein, and vitamins

Cooking Time: 12 minutes

Nourishing Lunche Recipes

1: Salmon and Quinoa Stuffed Bell Peppers:

Ingredients:2 bell peppers, halved

6 ounces salmon fillet, cooked and flaked

1/2 cup cooked quinoa

1/4 cup diced tomatoes

1 tablespoon chopped fresh parsley

Nutritional Value: Omega-3, protein, and fiber

Cooking Time: 25 minutes

2: Veggie and Lentil Soup:

Ingredients:1/2 cup dried green lentils

1 cup mixed vegetables (carrots, celery, spinach)

1/4 cup diced onions

4 cups low-sodium vegetable broth

1 teaspoon olive oil

Nutritional Value: Protein, fiber, and vitamins

Cooking Time: 30 minutes

3: Chicken and Avocado Lettuce Wraps:

Ingredients:4 large lettuce leaves

3 ounces grilled chicken breast, sliced

1/2 avocado, diced
1/4 cup cherry tomatoes, halved
Nutritional Value: Lean protein, healthy fats, and vitamins

4: **Cauliflower Rice and Shrimp Stir-Fry:**

Ingredients:1 cup cauliflower rice
6 ounces shrimp, peeled and deveined
1/2 cup broccoli florets
1/4 cup bell peppers, sliced
2 tablespoons low-sodium soy sauce
Nutritional Value: Low in carbs, high in protein and fiber
Cooking Time: 15 minutes

5: **Turkey and Vegetable Skewers:**

Ingredients:4 ounces turkey breast, cut into cubes
1/2 cup cherry tomatoes
1/2 cup bell peppers, sliced
Olive oil and herbs for marinade
Nutritional Value: Lean protein, vitamins, and antioxidants
Cooking Time: 20 minutes (including marinating and grilling)

6: **Spinach and Feta Stuffed Chicken Breast:**

Ingredients:2 boneless, skinless chicken breasts

1 cup fresh spinach
1/4 cup feta cheese, crumbled
1 teaspoon olive oil
Nutritional Value: Protein, vitamins, and healthy fats
Cooking Time: 25 minutes

7: **Cabbage** and Turkey Meatball Soup:
Ingredients:1/2 cup lean ground turkey
1 cup shredded cabbage
1/4 cup diced carrots
4 cups low-sodium chicken broth
1/2 teaspoon Italian seasoning
Nutritional Value: Protein, fiber, and vitamins
Cooking Time: 30 minutes
8: **Zucchini** Noodles with Pesto and Cherry Tomatoes:
Ingredients:2 medium zucchinis, spiralized
1/4 cup homemade basil pesto
1/2 cup cherry tomatoes, halved
1 tablespoon grated Parmesan cheese
Nutritional Value: Low in carbs, high in vitamins and healthy fats
Cooking Time: 15 minutes

9: **Mediterranean** Chickpea Salad:
Ingredients:1 can (15 oz) chickpeas, rinsed and drained

1/2 cup cucumber, diced

1/4 cup Kalamata olives, sliced

1/4 cup feta cheese, crumbled

Lemon vinaigrette for dressing

Nutritional Value: Protein, fiber, and antioxidants

10: **Cajun Shrimp and Quinoa Bowl:**

Ingredients:6 ounces shrimp, peeled and deveined

1/2 cup cooked quinoa

1/4 cup bell peppers, diced

Cajun seasoning for flavor

Nutritional Value: Protein, fiber, and vitamins

Cooking Time: 20 minutes

11: **Turkey and Quinoa Stuffed Peppers:**

Ingredients:2 bell peppers, halved

1/2 cup cooked quinoa

4 ounces ground turkey

1/4 cup diced tomatoes

Nutritional Value: Protein, fiber, and vitamins

Cooking Time: 30 minutes

12: **Broccoli and Chicken Stir-Fry:**

Ingredients:6 ounces chicken breast, sliced

1 cup broccoli florets

1/4 cup bell peppers, sliced
2 tablespoons low-sodium soy sauce
Nutritional Value: Protein, fiber, and antioxidants
Cooking Time: 15 minutes

13: **Cauliflower and Chickpea Salad:**

Ingredients:1 cup cauliflower florets, steamed
1/2 cup canned chickpeas, rinsed and drained
1/4 cup red onions, finely chopped
Lemon-tahini dressing for flavor
Nutritional Value: Low in carbs, high in fiber and protein

14: **Salmon and Avocado Quinoa Bowl:**

Ingredients:6 ounces grilled salmon fillet
1/2 cup cooked quinoa
1/4 cup diced avocado
1/4 cup cherry tomatoes, halved
Nutritional Value: Omega-3, protein, and healthy fats
Cooking Time: 20 minutes

15: **Greek Chicken Wrap:**

Ingredients:1 whole-grain wrap
4 ounces grilled chicken breast, sliced
1/4 cup cucumber, diced

2 tablespoons tzatziki sauce
Nutritional Value: Lean protein, vitamins, and probiotics

16: **Shrimp and Vegetable Brown Rice Bowl:**

Ingredients:6 ounces shrimp, peeled and deveined
1/2 cup cooked brown rice
1/4 cup broccoli florets
1/4 cup snow peas, sliced
Nutritional Value: Protein, fiber, and vitamins
Cooking Time: 15 minutes

17: **Eggplant and Tomato Quinoa Salad:**

Ingredients:1 cup cooked quinoa
1 cup eggplant, diced
1/2 cup cherry tomatoes, halved
2 tablespoons balsamic vinaigrette
Nutritional Value: High in fiber, vitamins, and antioxidants
Cooking Time: 20 minutes

18: **Cajun Black Bean and Turkey Chili:**

Ingredients:1/2 cup lean ground turkey
1 cup black beans, canned and rinsed
1/4 cup bell peppers, diced
Cajun seasoning for flavor

Nutritional Value: Protein, fiber, and antioxidants
Cooking Time: 30 minutes

19: **Mushroom and Spinach Quiche with Almond Flour Crust:**
Ingredients:1 cup almond flour
4 eggs
1 cup mushrooms, sliced
1 cup fresh spinach
Nutritional Value: Low in carbs, high in protein and healthy fats
Cooking Time: 35 minutes
20: Turkey and Vegetable Skillet with Cauliflower Rice:
Ingredients:1 cup cauliflower rice
4 ounces ground turkey
1/4 cup bell peppers, diced
1/4 cup zucchini, sliced
Nutritional Value: Lean protein, vitamins, and low in carbs
Cooking Time: 20 minutes

21: **Mediterranean Chickpea and Spinach Wrap:**
Ingredients:1 whole-grain wrap
1/2 cup canned chickpeas, rinsed and drained
1 cup fresh spinach

1/4 cup cherry tomatoes, halved
Nutritional Value: Protein, fiber, and vitamins

22: **Sesame Ginger Tofu Stir-Fry:**
Ingredients:1 cup tofu, cubed
1/2 cup broccoli florets
1/4 cup bell peppers, sliced
1 tablespoon low-sodium soy sauce
Nutritional Value: Protein, fiber, and antioxidants
Cooking Time: 15 minutes

23: **Chicken and Vegetable Zoodle Bowl:**
Ingredients:6 ounces grilled chicken breast, sliced
1 cup zucchini noodles (zoodles)
1/4 cup cherry tomatoes, halved
1 tablespoon olive oil
Nutritional Value: Lean protein, low in carbs, and vitamins
Cooking Time: 20 minutes

24: **Cabbage and Turkey Sausage Stir-Fry:**
Ingredients:1 cup shredded cabbage
2 turkey sausage links, sliced
1/4 cup bell peppers, julienned
1 tablespoon sesame oil

Nutritional Value: Low in carbs, high in fiber and protein
Cooking Time: 15 minutes

25: Lemon Herb Baked Cod with Quinoa:

Ingredients:6 ounces cod fillet

1/2 cup cooked quinoa

1 tablespoon fresh lemon juice

1 teaspoon mixed herbs (such as thyme and rosemary)

Nutritional Value: Omega-3, protein, and vitamins

Cooking Time: 25 minutes

26: Quinoa and Black Bean Stuffed Bell Peppers:

Ingredients:2 bell peppers, halved

1/2 cup cooked quinoa

1/2 cup black beans, canned and rinsed

1/4 cup diced tomatoes

Nutritional Value: Protein, fiber, and vitamins

Cooking Time: 30 minutes

27: Turkey and Vegetable Lettuce Wraps:

Ingredients:4 large lettuce leaves

3 ounces ground turkey

1/4 cup bell peppers, diced

1/4 cup shredded carrots
Nutritional Value: Lean protein, vitamins, and minerals
Cooking Time: 15 minutes

28: **Salmon and Avocado Salad:**

Ingredients:6 ounces grilled salmon fillet, flaked
2 cups mixed greens (lettuce, arugula)
1/2 avocado, sliced
1/4 cup cucumber, sliced
Nutritional Value: Omega-3, vitamins, and fiber

29: **Cauliflower and Chickpea Curry Bowl:**

Ingredients:1 cup cauliflower florets
1/2 cup cooked chickpeas
1/4 cup diced tomatoes
1/4 cup coconut milk
Nutritional Value: Low in carbs, high in fiber and protein
Cooking Time: 25 minutes

30: **Mushroom and Spinach Frittata:**

Ingredients:4 eggs
1 cup sliced mushrooms
1 cup fresh spinach
1/4 cup feta cheese, crumbled

Nutritional Value: Protein, vitamins, and healthy fats

Cooking Time: 20 minutes

31: **Baked Cod with Lemon Herb Quinoa:**

Ingredients:6 ounces cod fillet

1/2 cup cooked quinoa

1 tablespoon fresh lemon juice

1 teaspoon mixed herbs (such as thyme and rosemary)

Nutritional Value: Omega-3, protein, and vitamins

Cooking Time: 25 minutes

32: **Vegetarian Eggplant and Chickpea Stir-Fry:**

Ingredients:1 cup eggplant, diced

1/2 cup cooked chickpeas

1/4 cup bell peppers, sliced

2 tablespoons low-sodium soy sauce

Nutritional Value: Protein, fiber, and antioxidants

Cooking Time: 20 minutes

32: **Turkey and Spinach Stuffed Portobello Mushrooms:**

Ingredients:2 large portobello mushrooms

1/2 cup lean ground turkey

1 cup fresh spinach

1/4 cup mozzarella cheese, shredded
Nutritional Value: Protein, vitamins, and minerals
Cooking Time: 25 minutes

33: **Greek Quinoa Salad with Grilled Chicken:**

Ingredients:6 ounces grilled chicken breast, sliced
1/2 cup cooked quinoa
1/4 cup cherry tomatoes, halved
2 tablespoons feta cheese, crumbled
Nutritional Value: Protein, fiber, and antioxidants

34: **Cabbage and Shrimp Stir-Fry:**

Ingredients:1 cup shredded cabbage
6 ounces shrimp, peeled and deveined
1/4 cup snow peas, sliced
1 tablespoon sesame oil
Nutritional Value: Protein, vitamins, and low in carbs
Cooking Time: 15 minutes

35: **Turkey and Vegetable Quinoa Skillet:**

Ingredients:4 ounces lean ground turkey
1/2 cup cooked quinoa
1/4 cup bell peppers, diced

1/4 cup zucchini, sliced
Nutritional Value: Lean protein, fiber, and vitamins
Cooking Time: 20 minutes

36: **Vegetarian Lentil Soup:**

Ingredients:1/2 cup dried green lentils
1 cup mixed vegetables (carrots, celery, spinach)
1/4 cup diced onions
4 cups low-sodium vegetable broth
Nutritional Value: Protein, fiber, and vitamins
Cooking Time: 30 minutes

37: **Salmon and Cucumber Avocado Rolls:**

Ingredients:6 ounces smoked salmon
1/2 cucumber, julienned
1/2 avocado, sliced
Greek yogurt and dill sauce for dipping
Nutritional Value: Omega-3, fiber, and healthy fats

38: **Cauliflower and Chickpea Buddha Bowl:**

Ingredients:1 cup roasted cauliflower florets
1/2 cup cooked chickpeas
1/4 cup quinoa, cooked

1/4 cup shredded carrots

Nutritional Value: Fiber, protein, and vitamins

Cooking Time: 25 minutes

39: **Tomato Basil Zoodle Salad with Grilled Chicken:**

Ingredients:6 ounces grilled chicken breast, sliced

1 cup zucchini noodles (zoodles)

1/2 cup cherry tomatoes, halved

Fresh basil leaves, chopped

Nutritional Value: Lean protein, low in carbs, and antioxidants

40: **Egg Salad Lettuce Wraps:**

Ingredients:4 hard-boiled eggs, chopped

1/4 cup celery, finely diced

1 tablespoon mayonnaise (use a light version)

Lettuce leaves for wrapping

Nutritional Value: Protein, vitamins, and healthy fats

41: **Spaghetti Squash Primavera with Shrimp:**

Ingredients:1 medium spaghetti squash, cooked and shredded

6 ounces shrimp, peeled and deveined

1/2 cup cherry tomatoes, halved
1/4 cup bell peppers, sliced
Nutritional Value: Low in carbs, high in protein, and vitamins
Cooking Time: 30 minutes

41: **Turkey and Kale Stuffed Peppers:**

Ingredients:2 bell peppers, halved
1/2 cup lean ground turkey
1 cup kale, chopped
1/4 cup diced tomatoes
Nutritional Value: Lean protein, fiber, and vitamins
Cooking Time: 25 minutes

42: **Salmon and Vegetable Foil Packets:**

Ingredients:6 ounces salmon fillet
1/2 cup broccoli florets
1/4 cup bell peppers, sliced
1 tablespoon olive oil
Nutritional Value: Omega-3, vitamins, and minerals
Cooking Time: 20 minutes

43: **Spinach and Mushroom Omelette:**

Ingredients:2 eggs
1 cup fresh spinach
1/2 cup sliced mushrooms
1/4 cup shredded low-fat cheese

Nutritional Value: Protein, vitamins, and calcium
Cooking Time: 10 minutes

44: **Cabbage and Turkey Sausage Casserole:**

Ingredients:1 cup shredded cabbage
2 turkey sausage links, sliced
1/4 cup diced onions
1/4 teaspoon paprika
Nutritional Value: Low in carbs, high in fiber and protein
Cooking Time: 25 minutes

45: **Mediterranean Chickpea and Artichoke Salad:**

Ingredients:1/2 cup canned chickpeas, rinsed and drained
1/4 cup artichoke hearts, chopped
1/4 cup cherry tomatoes, halved
2 tablespoons feta cheese, crumbled
Nutritional Value: Protein, fiber, and antioxidants

46: **Shrimp and Broccoli Quinoa Bowl:**
Ingredients:
6 ounces shrimp, peeled and deveined
1/2 cup cooked quinoa
1 cup broccoli florets

1 tablespoon olive oil
Nutritional Value: Protein, fiber, and vitamins
Cooking Time: 15 minutes

47: **Turkey and Vegetable Lettuce Cups:**
Ingredients:
4 large lettuce leaves
4 ounces ground turkey
1/4 cup bell peppers, diced
1/4 cup carrots, shredded
Nutritional Value: Lean protein, vitamins, and minerals
Cooking Time: 20 minutes

48: **Mediterranean Chicken and Couscous Salad:**
Ingredients:
6 ounces grilled chicken breast, sliced
1/2 cup cooked whole-grain couscous
1/4 cup cherry tomatoes, halved
2 tablespoons feta cheese, crumbled
Nutritional Value: Protein, fiber, and antioxidants
49: Cauliflower and Chickpea Patties:
Ingredients:
1 cup cauliflower, grated
1/2 cup canned chickpeas, mashed
2 tablespoons almond flour

1 teaspoon cumin
Nutritional Value: Low in carbs, high in fiber and protein
Cooking Time: 25 minutes

50: **Asian Tofu and Vegetable Stir-Fry:**
Ingredients:
1 cup tofu, cubed
1/2 cup snap peas, sliced
1/4 cup bell peppers, julienned
1 tablespoon low-sodium soy sauce
Nutritional Value: Protein, fiber, and antioxidants
Cooking Time: 15 minutes

Dinners Recipes

1: **Grilled Lemon Herb Chicken:**
Ingredients:
2 boneless, skinless chicken breasts
2 tablespoons fresh lemon juice
1 tablespoon olive oil
1 teaspoon dried herbs (rosemary, thyme)

Nutritional Value: Lean protein, vitamins, and healthy fats
Cooking Time: 20 minutes

2: Vegetarian Cauliflower Fried Rice:
Ingredients:
1 cup cauliflower rice
1/4 cup diced carrots
1/4 cup peas
2 tablespoons low-sodium soy sauce
Nutritional Value: Low in carbs, fiber, and vitamins
Cooking Time: 15 minutes

3: Salmon and Asparagus Foil Packets:
Ingredients:
2 salmon fillets
1 cup asparagus, trimmed
1 tablespoon olive oil
Lemon slices for flavor
Nutritional Value: Omega-3, protein, and vitamins
Cooking Time: 25 minutes

4: Turkey and Vegetable Quinoa Skillet:
Ingredients:
4 ounces lean ground turkey
1/2 cup cooked quinoa
1/4 cup bell peppers, diced
1/4 cup zucchini, sliced
Nutritional Value: Lean protein, fiber, and vitamins

Cooking Time: 20 minutes

5: **Eggplant and Chickpea Curry:**

Ingredients:

1 cup eggplant, diced

1/2 cup canned chickpeas, rinsed and drained

1/4 cup diced tomatoes

1 tablespoon curry powder

Nutritional Value: Protein, fiber, and antioxidants

Cooking Time: 25 minutes

6: **Baked Cod with Tomato and Olive Relish:**

Ingredients:

6 ounces cod fillet

1/2 cup cherry tomatoes, diced

2 tablespoons Kalamata olives, sliced

1 tablespoon olive oil

Nutritional Value: Omega-3, protein, and healthy fats

Cooking Time: 20 minutes

7: **Mushroom and Spinach Stuffed Bell Peppers:**

Ingredients:

2 bell peppers, halved

1 cup sliced mushrooms

1 cup fresh spinach

1/4 cup feta cheese, crumbled

Nutritional Value: Protein, vitamins, and healthy fats

Cooking Time: 30 minutes

8: **Cajun Shrimp and Zucchini Noodles:**
Ingredients:
6 ounces shrimp, peeled and deveined
1 cup zucchini noodles (zoodles)
1/4 cup cherry tomatoes, halved
Cajun seasoning for flavor
Nutritional Value: Protein, low in carbs, and vitamins
Cooking Time: 15 minutes

9: **Quinoa and Black Bean Stuffed Peppers:**
Ingredients:
2 bell peppers, halved
1/2 cup cooked quinoa
1/2 cup black beans, canned and rinsed
1/4 cup diced tomatoes
Nutritional Value: Protein, fiber, and vitamins
Cooking Time: 30 minutes

10: **Greek Chicken Souvlaki Skewers:**
Ingredients:
6 ounces chicken breast, cut into cubes
1/4 cup plain Greek yogurt
1 teaspoon lemon juice
1 teaspoon dried oregano
Nutritional Value: Lean protein, probiotics, and vitamins

Cooking Time: 20 minutes (including marinating and grillings)

11: **Lemon Garlic Turkey Stir-Fry:**

Ingredients:

4 ounces lean ground turkey

1 cup broccoli florets

1/4 cup bell peppers, sliced

1 tablespoon olive oil

1 teaspoon minced garlic

Nutritional Value: Lean protein, fiber, and vitamins

Cooking Time: 15 minutes

12: **Mediterranean Baked Chicken Thighs:**

Ingredients:

2 chicken thighs, bone-in, skinless

1 tablespoon olive oil

1 teaspoon dried oregano

1/2 teaspoon garlic powder

1/4 cup cherry tomatoes, halved

Nutritional Value: Protein, healthy fats, and vitamins

Cooking Time: 30 minutes

13: **Cauliflower and Broccoli Gratin:**

Ingredients:

1 cup cauliflower florets

1 cup broccoli florets

1/4 cup grated Parmesan cheese
1/4 cup almond flour
1/2 cup unsweetened almond milk
Nutritional Value: Low in carbs, fiber, and calcium
Cooking Time: 25 minutes

14: Spaghetti Squash with Turkey Bolognese:
Ingredients:
1 small spaghetti squash
4 ounces lean ground turkey
1/2 cup diced tomatoes
1/4 cup tomato sauce (low-sugar)
Nutritional Value: Low in carbs, protein, and vitamins
Cooking Time: 40 minutes

15: Chickpea and Vegetable Curry:
Ingredients:
1 cup canned chickpeas, rinsed and drained
1 cup mixed vegetables (carrots, peas, bell peppers)
1/4 cup diced onions
1 tablespoon curry powder
Nutritional Value: Protein, fiber, and antioxidants
Cooking Time: 20 minutes

16: Mediterranean Chickpea and Spinach Stew:
Ingredients:
1/2 cup dried chickpeas, soaked and cooked
1 cup fresh spinach

1/4 cup cherry tomatoes, halved
1/4 cup red onion, diced
Nutritional Value: Protein, fiber, and antioxidants
Cooking Time: 30 minutes

17: Lemon Garlic Chicken with Brussels Sprouts:
Ingredients:
2 boneless, skinless chicken breasts
1 cup Brussels sprouts, halved
1 tablespoon olive oil
1 tablespoon fresh lemon juice
Nutritional Value: Lean protein, vitamins, and healthy fats
Cooking Time: 25 minutes
18: Cauliflower and Broccoli Gratin:
Ingredients:
1 cup cauliflower florets
1 cup broccoli florets
1/4 cup grated Parmesan cheese
1/2 cup unsweetened almond milk
Nutritional Value: Low in carbs, fiber, and vitamins
Cooking Time: 30 minutes

19: Shrimp and Vegetable Stir-Fry:
Ingredients:
6 ounces shrimp, peeled and deveined
1/2 cup bell peppers, sliced
1/2 cup snap peas, trimmed
1 tablespoon low-sodium soy sauce

Nutritional Value: Protein, vitamins, and antioxidants
Cooking Time: 15 minutes

20: Turkey and Quinoa Stuffed Acorn Squash:
Ingredients:
1 acorn squash, halved
4 ounces ground turkey
1/2 cup cooked quinoa
1/4 cup diced apples
Nutritional Value: Lean protein, fiber, and vitamins
Cooking Time: 40 minutes

21: Salmon and Quinoa Stuffed Bell Peppers:
Ingredients:
2 bell peppers, halved
6 ounces baked or grilled salmon, flaked
1/2 cup cooked quinoa
1/4 cup diced tomatoes
Nutritional Value: Omega-3, protein, and fiber
Cooking Time: 30 minutes

22: Vegetarian Lentil and Vegetable Soup:
Ingredients:
1/2 cup dried green lentils
1 cup mixed vegetables (carrots, celery, spinach)
1/4 cup diced onions
4 cups low-sodium vegetable broth
Nutritional Value: Protein, fiber, and vitamins

Cooking Time: 30 minutes

23: Chicken and Broccoli Almond Stir-Fry:
Ingredients:
6 ounces chicken breast, sliced
1 cup broccoli florets
1/4 cup sliced almonds
1 tablespoon low-sodium soy sauce
Nutritional Value: Lean protein, fiber, and healthy fats
Cooking Time: 20 minutes

24: Eggplant and Tomato Bake:
Ingredients:
1 large eggplant, sliced
1 cup cherry tomatoes, halved
2 tablespoons olive oil
1 teaspoon dried basil
Nutritional Value: Low in carbs, fiber, and vitamins
Cooking Time: 25 minutes
25: Mushroom and Spinach Stuffed Chicken Thighs:
Ingredients:
4 boneless, skinless chicken thighs
1 cup sliced mushrooms
1 cup fresh spinach
1/4 cup feta cheese, crumbled
Nutritional Value: Protein, vitamins, and healthy fats

Cooking Time: 30 minutes

26: Turkey and Vegetable Zucchini Boats:
Ingredients:
2 medium zucchini
4 ounces ground turkey
1/4 cup bell peppers, diced
1/4 cup tomato sauce (low-sugar)
Nutritional Value: Lean protein, fiber, and vitamins
Cooking Time: 25 minutes

27: Cauliflower and Chickpea Curry Bowl:
Ingredients:
1 cup cauliflower florets
1/2 cup cooked chickpeas
1/4 cup diced tomatoes
1/4 cup coconut milk
Nutritional Value: Low in carbs, high in fiber, and protein
Cooking Time: 25 minutes

28: Grilled Lemon Garlic Shrimp Skewers:
Ingredients:
6 ounces shrimp, peeled and deveined
1 tablespoon olive oil
1 tablespoon fresh lemon juice
1 teaspoon minced garlic
Nutritional Value: Protein, vitamins, and healthy fats

Cooking Time: 15 minutes (including marinating and grilling)

29: Chicken and Vegetable Skillet with Quinoa:
Ingredients:
6 ounces grilled chicken breast, sliced
1/2 cup bell peppers, sliced
1/4 cup cherry tomatoes, halved
1/2 cup cooked quinoa
Nutritional Value: Lean protein, fiber, and vitamins
Cooking Time: 20 minutes

30: Salmon and Asparagus Sheet Pan Dinner:
Ingredients:
2 salmon fillets
1 bunch asparagus, trimmed
1 tablespoon olive oil
Lemon wedges for serving
Nutritional Value: Omega-3, protein, and vitamins
Cooking Time: 25 minutes

31: Vegetarian Stuffed Bell Peppers:
Ingredients:
2 bell peppers, halved
1/2 cup cooked brown rice
1/2 cup black beans, canned and rinsed
1/4 cup diced tomatoes
Nutritional Value: Fiber, protein, and vitamins

Cooking Time: 30 minutes

32: Turkey and Vegetable Lettuce Wraps:
Ingredients:
1 pound ground turkey
1/2 cup diced bell peppers
1/4 cup shredded carrots
1/4 cup hoisin sauce
Nutritional Value: Lean protein, fiber, and vitamins
Cooking Time: 20 minutes

33: Eggplant Lasagna:
Ingredients:
1 large eggplant, sliced
1 cup ricotta cheese
1/2 cup marinara sauce (low-sugar)
1/4 cup grated Parmesan cheese
Nutritional Value: Low in carbs, protein, and vitamins
Cooking Time: 40 minutes

34: Shrimp and Avocado Salad Bowl:
Ingredients:
6 ounces grilled shrimp
1/2 avocado, sliced
1 cup mixed greens (lettuce, spinach)
Balsamic vinaigrette for dressing
Nutritional Value: Protein, healthy fats, and vitamins

35: Grilled Chicken and Vegetable Skewers:
Ingredients:
6 ounces chicken breast, cut into cubes
1/2 cup cherry tomatoes
1/2 cup bell peppers, sliced
1/4 cup red onion, diced
Nutritional Value: Lean protein, vitamins, and antioxidants
Cooking Time: 20 minutes (including marinating and grilling)

36: Quinoa and Black Bean Stuffed Zucchini:
Ingredients:
2 medium zucchini
1/2 cup cooked quinoa
1/2 cup black beans, canned and rinsed
1/4 cup diced tomatoes
Nutritional Value: Protein, fiber, and vitamins
Cooking Time: 25 minutes

37: Mushroom and Spinach Omelette:
Ingredients:
3 eggs
1/2 cup sliced mushrooms
1 cup fresh spinach
1/4 cup feta cheese, crumbled
Nutritional Value: Protein, vitamins, and healthy fats

Cooking Time: 15 minutes

38: Baked Cod with Mediterranean Salsa:
Ingredients:
2 cod fillets
1/2 cup cherry tomatoes, diced
2 tablespoons Kalamata olives, sliced
1 tablespoon olive oil
Nutritional Value: Omega-3, protein, and healthy fats
Cooking Time: 20 minutes

39: Turkey and Vegetable Stir-Fry:
Ingredients:
4 ounces ground turkey
1/2 cup broccoli florets
1/4 cup bell peppers, sliced
1/4 cup snow peas
Nutritional Value: Lean protein, fiber, and vitamins
Cooking Time: 20 minutes

40: Cauliflower and Broccoli Grilled Skewers:
Ingredients:
1 cup cauliflower florets
1 cup broccoli florets
1/4 cup olive oil
1 teaspoon garlic powder
Nutritional Value: Low in carbs, fiber, and vitamins

Cooking Time: 15 minutes (including marinating and grilling)

41: Lemon Herb Baked Chicken Thighs:
Ingredients:
4 bone-in, skinless chicken thighs
1 tablespoon olive oil
1 tablespoon fresh lemon juice
1 teaspoon dried herbs (thyme, rosemary)
Nutritional Value: Lean protein, vitamins, and healthy fats
Cooking Time: 35 minutes

42: Vegetarian Eggplant and Chickpea Casserole:
Ingredients:
1 large eggplant, sliced
1 cup canned chickpeas, rinsed and drained
1/2 cup diced tomatoes
1/4 cup feta cheese, crumbled
Nutritional Value: Protein, fiber, and vitamins
Cooking Time: 40 minutes

43: Turkey and Spinach Stuffed Portobello Mushrooms:
Ingredients:
4 large Portobello mushrooms
8 ounces ground turkey
1 cup fresh spinach
1/4 cup grated Parmesan cheese

Nutritional Value: Lean protein, vitamins, and healthy fats
Cooking Time: 25 minutes

44: Salmon and Asparagus Quinoa Bowl:
Ingredients:
6 ounces grilled salmon fillet
1/2 cup cooked quinoa
1 cup asparagus, trimmed
Lemon-tahini dressing for flavor
Nutritional Value: Omega-3, protein, and fiber
Cooking Time: 20 minutes

45:Grilled Lemon Herb Chicken Breast:
Ingredients:
2 boneless, skinless chicken breasts
1 tablespoon olive oil
1 tablespoon fresh lemon juice
1 teaspoon dried herbs (oregano, thyme)
Nutritional Value: Lean protein, vitamins, and healthy fats
Cooking Time: 20 minutes

46: Zucchini Noodles with Pesto and Cherry Tomatoes:
Ingredients:
2 medium zucchinis, spiralized
2 tablespoons basil pesto
1/2 cup cherry tomatoes, halved

1 tablespoon pine nuts (optional)

Nutritional Value: Low in carbs, healthy fats, and vitamins

Cooking Time: 15 minutes

47: Stir-Fried Tofu and Broccoli:

Ingredients:

1 cup tofu, cubed

1 cup broccoli florets

1/4 cup low-sodium soy sauce

1 tablespoon sesame oil

Nutritional Value: Plant-based protein, fiber, and vitamins

Cooking Time: 20 minutes

48: Cabbage and Turkey Meatball Soup:

Ingredients:

1/2 head cabbage, shredded

8 ounces ground turkey

1/4 cup diced onions

4 cups low-sodium chicken broth

Nutritional Value: Lean protein, fiber, and vitamins

Cooking Time: 30 minutes

49: Mushroom and Spinach Stuffed Chicken Breast:

Ingredients:

2 boneless, skinless chicken breasts

1 cup sliced mushrooms

1 cup fresh spinach

1/4 cup feta cheese, crumbled
Nutritional Value: Lean protein, vitamins, and healthy fats
Cooking Time: 25 minutes

50: Spaghetti Squash Primavera:
Ingredients:
1 medium spaghetti squash
1/2 cup cherry tomatoes, halved
1/2 cup broccoli florets
1/4 cup grated Parmesan cheese
Nutritional Value: Low in carbs, fiber, and vitamins
Cooking Time: 40 minutes

Snacks and Smoothies

Snacks:

1: **Greek Yogurt Parfait:**
Ingredients:
1/2 cup Greek yogurt
1/4 cup mixed berries (blueberries, strawberries)
1 tablespoon chopped nuts (almonds or walnuts)

1 teaspoon honey (optional)

Nutritional Value: Protein, antioxidants, and healthy fats

2:Veggie Sticks with Hummus:

Ingredients:

1 cup assorted veggie sticks (carrots, cucumber, bell peppers)

2 tablespoons hummus

Nutritional Value: Fiber, vitamins, and healthy fats

3: Cheese and Whole Grain Crackers:

Ingredients:

1 ounce low-fat cheese

10 whole grain crackers

Nutritional Value: Protein, fiber, and calcium

4: Hard-Boiled Egg and Avocado Slices:

Ingredients:

1 hard-boiled egg

1/2 avocado, sliced

Sprinkle of salt and pepper

Nutritional Value: Protein, healthy fats, and vitamins

5: Cucumber and Smoked Salmon Roll-Ups:

Ingredients:

4 cucumber slices

2 ounces smoked salmon

1 tablespoon cream cheese
Nutritional Value: Omega-3, protein, and vitamins

Smoothies:

6: **Berry Blast Smoothie:**
Ingredients:
1/2 cup mixed berries (strawberries, blueberries, raspberries)
1/2 cup unsweetened almond milk
1/2 cup Greek yogurt
1 tablespoon chia seeds
Nutritional Value: Antioxidants, protein, and fiber

7: **Green Power Smoothie:**
Ingredients:
1 cup spinach leaves
1/2 banana
1/2 cup pineapple chunks
1/2 cup coconut water
Nutritional Value: Vitamins, potassium, and fiber

8: **Cinnamon Apple Pie Smoothie:**
Ingredients:
1 medium apple, peeled and diced
1/2 cup plain Greek yogurt
1/2 teaspoon cinnamon
1/2 cup unsweetened almond milk
Nutritional Value: Fiber, protein, and antioxidants

9: **Mango and Ginger Smoothie:**
Ingredients:
1 cup mango chunks
1/2 teaspoon grated ginger
1/2 cup plain Greek yogurt
1/2 cup water or coconut water
Nutritional Value: Vitamin C, probiotics, and anti-inflammatory properties

10: **Chocolate Avocado Protein Smoothie:**
Ingredients:
1/2 avocado
1 tablespoon cocoa powder (unsweetened)
1 scoop whey protein powder
1/2 cup unsweetened almond milk
Nutritional Value: Healthy fats, protein, and antioxidants

Snacks:

11: **Almond Butter and Banana Slices:**
Ingredients:
1 medium banana, sliced
2 tablespoons almond butter
Nutritional Value: Healthy fats, potassium, and protein

12: **Yogurt-Covered Blueberries:**

Ingredients:

1/2 cup fresh blueberries

2 tablespoons Greek yogurt (unsweetened)

1 teaspoon honey (optional)

Nutritional Value: Antioxidants, protein, and probiotics

13: **Spicy Edamame:**

Ingredients:

1 cup edamame (steamed)

1/2 teaspoon chili powder

1/2 teaspoon garlic powder

Nutritional Value: Protein, fiber, and vitamins

14: **Cherry Tomato and Mozzarella Skewers:**

Ingredients:

1 cup cherry tomatoes

1 ounce fresh mozzarella balls

Fresh basil leaves

Nutritional Value: Protein, antioxidants, and calcium

15: **Cottage Cheese and Pineapple Bowl:**

Ingredients:

1/2 cup low-fat cottage cheese

1/2 cup pineapple chunks

Sprinkle of cinnamon

Nutritional Value: Protein, vitamin C, and calcium

Smoothies:

16: **Peach and Kale Smoothie:**
Ingredients:
1 cup frozen peach slices
1 cup kale leaves, stems removed
1/2 banana
1/2 cup unsweetened almond milk
Nutritional Value: Vitamins, fiber, and antioxidants

17: **Minty Melon Smoothie:**
Ingredients:
1 cup honeydew melon, diced
1/2 cup cucumber, peeled and sliced
1/2 teaspoon fresh mint leaves
1/2 cup coconut water
Nutritional Value: Hydration, vitamins, and antioxidants

18: **Avocado and Berry Protein Smoothie:**
Ingredients:
1/2 avocado
1/2 cup mixed berries (strawberries, blueberries)
1 scoop plant-based protein powder
1/2 cup almond milk
Nutritional Value: Healthy fats, protein, and antioxidants

19: **Turmeric and Ginger Citrus Smoothie:**
Ingredients:
1/2 teaspoon ground turmeric

1/2 teaspoon grated ginger
Juice of 1 orange
1/2 cup plain Greek yogurt
Nutritional Value: Anti-inflammatory properties, vitamin C, and probiotics

20: **Vanilla Almond Protein Smoothie:**
Ingredients:
1 scoop vanilla protein powder
1 tablespoon almond butter
1/2 banana
1/2 cup unsweetened almond milk
Nutritional Value: Protein, healthy fats, and potassium

Snacks:

21: **Cherry Almond Energy Bites:**
Ingredients:
1/2 cup dried cherries
1/2 cup almonds
1 tablespoon chia seeds
1/2 teaspoon vanilla extract
Nutritional Value: Protein, healthy fats, and antioxidants

22: **Turkey and Cheese Roll-Ups:**
Ingredients:
4 slices low-sodium turkey breast
2 slices reduced-fat cheese
1/2 cucumber, julienned
Nutritional Value: Protein, calcium, and fiber

23: **Pistachio and Dark Chocolate Mix:**
Ingredients:
1/4 cup pistachios (unsalted)
1 tablespoon dark chocolate chips
1 tablespoon dried cranberries
Nutritional Value: Healthy fats, antioxidants, and fiber

24: **Avocado Tomato Salsa:**
Ingredients:
1 avocado, diced
1/2 cup cherry tomatoes, diced
1 tablespoon red onion, finely chopped
1 tablespoon lime juice
Nutritional Value: Healthy fats, vitamins, and fiber

25: **Cottage Cheese with Pineapple:**
Ingredients:
1/2 cup low-fat cottage cheese
1/2 cup fresh pineapple chunks
Sprinkle of cinnamon
Nutritional Value: Protein, vitamin C, and calcium

Smoothies:

26: **Strawberry Banana Protein Smoothie:**
Ingredients:
1/2 cup strawberries (fresh or frozen)
1/2 banana
1 scoop whey protein powder

1/2 cup unsweetened almond milk

Nutritional Value: Protein, vitamin C, and potassium

27: **Blueberry Avocado Green Smoothie:**

Ingredients:

1/2 cup blueberries (fresh or frozen)

1/4 avocado

Handful of spinach leaves

1/2 cup water or coconut water

Nutritional Value: Antioxidants, healthy fats, and vitamins

28: **Vanilla Almond Berry Smoothie Bowl:**

Ingredients:

1/2 cup mixed berries (strawberries, blueberries)

1/2 banana

1/2 cup Greek yogurt

1 tablespoon almond butter

Nutritional Value: Protein, antioxidants, and healthy fats

29: **Tropical Green Smoothie:**

Ingredients:

1/2 cup pineapple chunks

1/2 cup mango chunks

Handful of kale leaves

1/2 cup coconut water

Nutritional Value: Vitamins, fiber, and hydration

30: **Peach and Almond Butter Smoothie:**

Ingredients:

1 cup frozen peach slices

1 tablespoon almond butter

1/2 cup Greek yogurt

1/2 cup unsweetened almond milk

Nutritional Value: Protein, healthy fats, and vitamins

Conclusion

As you turn the final pages of your Diabetic Disease Cookbook for Women, reflect on the journey you've traversed—a journey overflowing with recipes that do more than tantalize your taste buds; they chart a course for sustained health and vitality. Every dish has been chosen with a singular purpose: to harmonize your blood sugar, boost your energy, and nourish your body in a way that's specifically curated for the unique challenges you face with diabetes.

You've been introduced to an array of meals—from morning starters that awaken your senses to lunches that keep you powered throughout your day, right down to dinners that wrap up your evenings with a sense of fulfillment. Your discovery that balanced snacks and sweets can coexist with a diabetes-aware diet proves that pleasure need not be sacrificed at the altar of health.

This is more than a cookbook; it's your blueprint for a transformative lifestyle shift, one that takes the profound wisdom of nutrition and translates it into a practical, everyday ritual. It's your toolkit for smart, savory choices that, meal by meal, day by day, rewrite your health narrative.

With this dietary transformation, you become a beacon of motivation, demonstrating the resilience and spirit of women facing diabetes. Your kitchen is now a cradle of change, where each recipe is a stride towards better well-being.

Consider this not a diet, but a new dialect in which to express self-love. Every ingredient you choose speaks of care, every dish you prepare articulates empowerment. Let these recipes be but the first words in the vibrant story of your own well-being.

Harness the power that lies within you. With each nutritious bite, craft a brighter tomorrow. Embrace this shift, letting your renewed food choices be the driving force behind a life brimming with health. Recall that your story of wellness is yours to write—do so boldly, celebrating each triumph along the way.

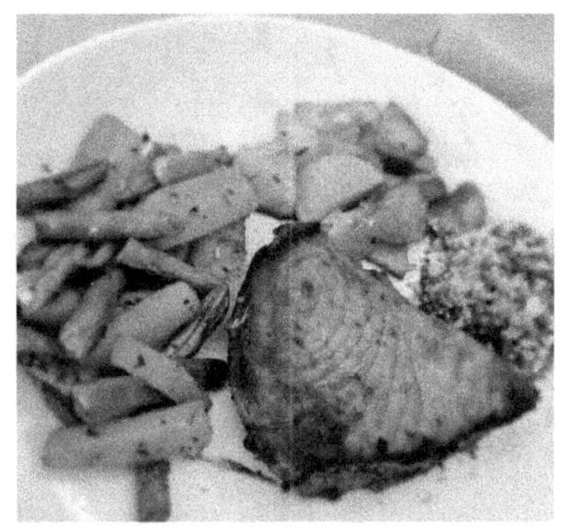

www.ingramcontent.com/pod-product-compliance
Lightning Source LLC
Chambersburg PA
CBHW071018260726

48662CB00022B/580